CHICKEN-

ACONITUM NAPELLUS

Early cases, with restlessness, anxiety and high fever.

ANTIMONIUM TARTARICUM

Delayed or receding, blue or pustular eruptions.
Drowsy, sweaty and relaxed; nausea.
Tardy eruption, to accelerate it.
Associated with bronchitis, especially in children. (*Ant. crud.*)

BELLADONNA

Severe headache: face flushed; hot skin.
Drowsiness with inability to sleep.

MERCURIUS

"Should vesicles suppurate."

RHUS TOXICODENDRON

Intense itching.
"Generally the only remedy required; under its action the disease soon disappears."

Supplied by
Ainsworths Homoeopathic Pharmacy
38 New Cavendish Street, London W1M 7LH
Tel: 071-935 5330   Fax: 071-486 4313

DIPHTHERIA

APIS

Throat bright-red, puffy, "varnished". Uvula long; œdematous. Nothing must touch throat (*Lach.*).

ARSENICUM ALBUM

Membrane looks dry, shrivelled. The *Arsenicum* anxiety, restlessness and prostration are present.
Worse at night: 1–2 a.m.
Chilliness: incessant thirst for small quantities.

BAPTISIA

Putridity: with dull red face; drowsiness; patient as if drugged.
Membrane dark: dry brown tongue.

DIPHTHERINUM

When the attack from the onset tends to malignancy.
Painless diphtheria. Symptoms almost, or entirely objective.
Patient weak, apathetic. Stupor.
Dark-red swelling of tonsils and throat.
Breath and discharges very offensive (*Merc. cy.*).
Membrane thick, dark-grey or brownish black.
Temperature low, or subnormal. Pulse weak and rapid. Vital reaction very low.
Epistaxis, or profound prostration from the onset. Collapse almost at the very beginning.
Swallows without pain, but fluids are vomited or returned through nose.
Laryngeal diphtheria; post-diphtheric paralysis. (*Caust.*, *Cocc.*, *Gels.* and *Lycopodium*.)
When the patient from the first seems doomed, and the most carefully-selected remedies fail to relieve, or permanently improve.
To remove persistent diphtheria-organisms, in "carriers".

Like all the nosodes, it is practically worthless below the 30th potency while its curative virtues increase with the higher potencies. It should not be repeated too frequently.

DIPHTHERIA

KALI BICHROMICUM
Nasal diphtheria: ropy discharges.
Exudation tough and firmly adherent.

LAC CANINUM
Patients nervous, imaginative, highly sensitive.
Skin hypersensitive (*Lach.*). Touch unbearable, though hard pressure gives no pain.
Membrane pearly, or silver white.
Milky coating on tongue.
Characteristic feature is *alternation of sides*.
Pain will jump back and forth from side to side.

LACHESIS MUTA
Membrane starts on left side, spreads to right.
Face and throat look cyanotic. Choking.
Cold things more easily swallowed than hot.
Great sensitiveness of neck and throat, so that patient cannot stand the touch of bedclothes, and pulls neck of night attire open.
General and local aggravation from heat, and all symptoms are worse after sleep. The longer the sleep, the worse he is on waking.
Characteristics are loquacity and suspicion.

LYCOPODIUM
Patient worse from 4 to 8 p.m.
Starts in nose (*Kali bic.*) or right side throat, spreads to left.
Warm drinks more easily swallowed: but reverse sometimes the case.
Movement of nostrils.
Diminished urine or copious sediment of urates, or fine red sand.

MERCURIUS CYANATUS
Fairly rapid onset, with prostration.
One or both sides of throat affected.
Membrane spreads rapidly over entire throat.
Colour white, yellow, or greenish.
Tongue thickly coated, moist; salivation.
Odour always putrid. Hot sweats.
Tepid liquids better swallowed than hot or cold.
Patient (generally) worse late evening and night.
Has also proved curative in Vincent's Angina.

PHYTOLACCA

Frequently indicated.

Membrane grey or white, may start on uvula.

May spread from right tonsil to left (*Lyc.*). But, unlike *Lyc.*, the pain is worse from heat.

Fauces dark-red: complains of lump in throat; or as if red-hot ball had stuck in throat.

Pain goes to ear.

ERYSIPELAS

ACONITUM NAPELLUS

Sudden violent onset after exposure to cold wind.
Intense fever, with restlessness, and *fear of death*.

APIS

May be in patches. Great tumefaction.
High degree of inflammation, with *stinging*, *burning*, and *œdema* and vesication.
Eyelids like sacs of water.
Amelioration from cold; aggravation from heat.
Fidgety, nervous, fretful: sleepless.

ARSENICUM ALBUM

"Sudden inflammatory conditions like gangrenous and erysipelatous inflammations.
A sudden inflammation that tends to produce malignancy in the part, belongs to *Arsenicum*."
The secretions of *Arsen.* are acrid.
Characteristic, *burnings relieved by heat*: intense *anxiety*, *restlessness* and prostration.

BAPTISIA

Drowsy, dusky, comatose; face dark-red, with besotted expression. May be roused, but falls asleep answering.
Typhoid conditions, in the course of disease.
Acts very rapidly; rapid collapse, and rapid restoration. (*Crot. h.*)

BELLADONNA

Swelling, smooth, bright-red, streaked red; or deep, dark red.
Not much tendency to œdema or vesication.
Pains are throbbing; throbbing in brain.
Brain affected. Cases with delirium.
Jerking of limbs.
Belladonna is acute, *sudden*, and violent.
Belladonna is red, and intensely hot, dry.

CANTHARIS

Erysipelas of face with large blisters.
Burning in eyes: whole atmosphere looks yellow: scalding tears.
Like *Rhus*, but when very violent, *Canth.* will be indicated.
"*Rhus* has the blisters and the burning, but in *Canth.* between your two visits the erysipelas has grown black: it is a dusky rapid change that has taken place, looks as if gangrene would set in. Burning like fire from touch: as if the finger were a coal of fire. Not so in *Rhus*.
"The little blisters, if touched, burn like fire. *Eruptions burn when touched*" (KENT).
Erysipelas of eyes, with gangrenous tendency. "Unquenchable thirst with disgust for drinks."

CROTALUS HORRIDUS

Frequently recurring erysipelas of face.
General local phlegmonous or œdematous erysipelas. Skin bluish-red; low fever.
Gangrene: skin separated from muscles by a fœtid fluid. Black spots with red areola and dark, blackish redness of adjacent tissues.
"*Crotalus* is indicated in disease of the very lowest, the most putrid type, coming on with unusual rapidity, reaching that putrid state in an unusually short time" (KENT). (*Bapt.*)

CROTON TIGLIUM

"*Erysipelas that itches very much.*"
"Eruptions that itch very much; but cannot bear to scratch, as it hurts. A very slight scratch, a mere rub, serves to allay the irritation" (GUERNSEY).
Sensation, "Insects creeping on face."
"Cough disappears and the eruption comes; then eruption goes and cough comes back."

CUPRUM METALLICUM

Erysipelas of face disappears suddenly.
Eruptions "strike in" and cramps, spasms, convulsions supervene. To bring the eruption back, with relief.
Cramps begin characteristically in fingers and toes.

EUPHORBIUM

Vesicular erysipelas: erysipelas bulbosum.
Red inflammatory swelling, with vesicles as large as peas, filled with yellow liquid.
Red, inflammatory swelling, with boring, grinding, gnawing from gums into ear, followed by itching and tingling.
Vesicles burst and emit a "yellow humour".
Shuddering and chilliness.
Temporary attacks of craziness.

HIPPOZÆNINUM
(Nosode of Glanders)

"Malignant erysipelas, particularly if attended by *large formation of pus, and destruction of parts.* Ulcers with no disposition to heal, livid appearance" (CLARKE).

LACHESIS MUTA

Purple, mottled, puffy.
"When the cerebral condition does not yield to *Belladonna.*" Bell. is red: *Lach. less red and more blue.*
Especially affects the left side.
Lachesis, typically, is worse after sleep: is loquacious—suspicious—jealous.
Is hypersensitive to touch, esp. on throat: wants face free, or suffocates.

MERCURIUS

With salivation: bitter or salt taste.
With offensiveness: breath, sweat.
Erysipelas with sloughing: with "brown mortification". With burning: ulceration.
Chilliness and heat alternately: or heat and shuddering at the same time.
Creeping chilliness: in single parts: in places of pus formation, or ulceration.
Worse at night.

RHUS TOXICODENDRON

Erysipelas of the vesicular variety, accompanied by *restlessness.*
Erysipelas of face with burning; large blisters, rapidly extending: becomes very purple and pits on pressure.
Often extends from l. to r. across face.
Rhus is worse from damp: from cold: relieved, temporarily, by motion.

SECALE CORNUTUM

Gangrenous erysipelas: competes with *Ars*. The only distinguishing feature between the two remedies may be that *Secale* wants cold and *Arsenicum* wants heat.

Burning: "sparks of fire" falling on the part.

Formication: "mice creeping under the skin."

THUJA

Œdematous erysipelas of face.

Cases that occur in the much vaccinated may need *Thuja*, or cases that occur *after vaccination*.

A curious, characteristic symptom, profuse sweat only on uncovered parts.

VERATRUM VIRIDE

"One peculiar symptom I have verified in a very severe case of erysipelas, which was accompanied by great delirium, is *a narrow, well-defined red streak right through the middle of the tongue*" (NASH).

"Phlegmonous erysipelas of face and head" (CLARKE).

LESS SEVERE CASES

AMMONIUM CARBONICUM

"Erysipelas of old, debilitated persons.

Eruption faintly developed, or has seemed to disappear, from weakness of patient's vitality to keep it on the surface.

With cerebral symptoms, simulating a drunken stupor" (NASH).

"Eruption comes out, and does not give relief to the patient."

"Erysipelas of old people when cerebral symptoms are developed."

Defective reaction.

ARNICA

"Erysipelas of face, with *soreness*, and sore *bruised feeling* all over the body: you need not wait longer before prescribing *Arnica*."

"Bed feels too hard: must move to get into a new place." "*Rhus* moves from restlessness and uneasiness, cannot lie still: *Arnica*, to ease the *soreness* by getting into a new place" (KENT).

GRAPHITES

"Eruptions oozing out a thick, honey-like fluid . . . erysipelas sometimes takes this form, and in such cases recurs again and again" (*Sulph.*).

Erysipelatous, moist, scurfy sores.

Or, "Thin, *sticky*, glutinous, transparent watery fluid" (GUERNSEY, *Keynotes*).

HEPAR SULPHURIS CALCAREA

Any trouble occurring on the skin, when there is *great sensitiveness to the slightest touch* (*Canth.*).

Extreme sensitiveness runs through the whole remedy: to the slightest draught of air: to the slightest noise: and also mental sensitiveness and irritability—almost to murder, when angered.

PULSATILLA

Erysipelas in the *typical Pulsatilla patient*.

Mild, but irritable: changeable: weeps: craves sympathy.

Craves open air: cool air: worse for heat. Not hungry or thirsty.

SULPHUR

Recurrent attacks of erysipelas (*Graph.*).

Much burning: worse from heat of bed or room. Purplish appearance (*Lach.*).

"For erysipelas, as a name, we have no remedy, but when a patient has erysipelas and his symptoms conform to those of *Sulphur*, you will cure him with *Sulph.*" (KENT).

"When symptoms agree, *Sulph.* will be found a curative medicine in erysipelas."

The typical *Sulph.* patient is hungry, especially at 10 to 11 a.m. Loves fat, "Eats anything."

Kicks off the clothes at night, or puts feet out. Craves, or hates, or is worse from fats.

His eruptions itch; are worse from heat, warm room, warm bed and from washing.

Worse at night. Skin cannot bear woollens.

The untidy ragged philosopher. Selfish.

"*Sulphur* may be given on a paucity of symptoms."

HERPES ZOSTER
(SHINGLES)

APIS
Burning and *stinging* pain, much swelling.
Vesicles large, sometimes confluent.
Come out in cold weather.
Ulcerate with great burning, stinging pain.
Worse warmth: better cold applications.

ARSENICUM ALBUM
Confluent herpetic eruptions with *intense burning* of the blisters.
Sleepless after midnight.
Nausea and prostration: weakness.
Worse from cold of any kind, better from warmth.
"Herpes having a red, unwholesome appearance."

MEZEREUM
With severe neuralgic pains.
Itching, after scratching, turns to burning.
Worse from touch: in bed.
Vesicles form a brownish scab.

RANUNCULUS BULBOSUS
One has over and over again seen shingles clear up rapidly with 2 or 3 doses of *Ran. b.* in high potency—10m.
Vesicles filled with thin, acrid fluid.
Burning-itching vesicles in clusters.
Worse from touch, motion, after eating.
Severe neuralgic pains, especially intercostal.

RHUS TOXICODENDRON
"Probably no remedy more often found useful in herpes zoster. Especially when it occurs after a wetting."

VARIOLINUM
BURNETT said *Variolinum* had wiped out the condition, pain and all—and one has seen this also.

MEASLES

ACONITUM NAPELLUS

Catarrh and high fever: before rash clinches diagnosis.
Redness conjunctivae: dry, barking cough.
Itching, burning skin: rash rough and miliary.
Restless, anxious, tossing: frightened.

BELLADONNA

Rash bright-red: skin hot and dry—such cases as suggest scarlet fever.

EUPHRASIA

Cases with great catarrhal intensity.
"A wonderful medicine in measles. When symptoms agree will make a violent attack of measles turn into a very simple form...
"Streaming, burning tears; photophobia; running from nose; intense, throbbing headache, dry cough and rash" (KENT).
Copious *acrid* lachrymation, with streaming, *bland* discharge from nose (rev. of *Allium cepa*, which has acrid discharge from nose, but bland from eyes).

GELSEMIUM

Chills and heats chase one another. Sneezing and sore throat: excoriating nasal discharge.
Severe, heavy headache: occipital pain.
Thirstlessness is the rule with *Gels.* (*Puls.*).
Drowsy and stupid. Lids heavy: eyes inflamed.
Face dark-red, swollen, besotted look (*Bapt.*).

KALI BICHROMICUM

"Is like *Puls.* only worse." Follows *Puls. Puls. in the mild cases.*
It has a rash like measles, with catarrh of eyes.
Measles with purulent discharge eyes and ears. With pustules on cornea.
Salivary glands swollen: catarrhal deafness.
Kali bich. has stringy, ropy discharges.

MORBILLINUM
Prophylactic for contacts.

PULSATILLA
"If much fever, *Puls.* will not be the remedy."
Catarrhal symptoms: profuse lachrymation.
Dry mouth, but seldom thirsty.

SULPHUR
"Measles with a purplish appearance. *Sulphur* to modify the case when the skin is dusky and the rash does not come out."
"The routinist can do pretty well in this disease with *Puls.* and *Sulph.*, occasionally requiring *Acon.* and *Euphrasia*" (KENT).
Convalescence slow, and the patient is weak and prostrate.

Tardy or Suppressed Eruption: Brain Affected
APIS
Rash goes in and brain symptoms appear.
Stupor with stinging pains, extorting cries (*Crie cerebrale*).
Thirstless: worse from heat, hot room, hot fire.
Better cool air. Urine scanty.
A great remedy for œdema and effusions.

BRYONIA ALBA
Rash tardy to appear.
Hard, dry cough with tearing pain.
Little or no expectoration.
Or rash disappears and child drowsy: pale, twitching face, chewing motion of jaws (*Zinc.* grits teeth).
Any motion causes child to scream with pain.
Mild delirium, "Wants to go home," when at home.
Or, instead of rash, bronchitis or pneumonia, with *Bry.* symptoms.

CUPRUM METALLICUM
Symptoms violent. Starts up from sleep.
Spasms: cramps: convulsions.
Cramps of fingers and toes, or start there.

MEASLES

HELLEBORUS NIGER

"When entire sensorial life is suspended, and child lies in profound stupor."

STRAMONIUM

Rash not out properly. Child hot, bright-red face. Tosses, cries as if frightened in sleep. Convulsive movements.

ZINCUM METALLICUM

Where child is too weak to develop eruption.
Rash comes out sparingly. Body rather cool.
Lies in stupor gritting teeth. (*Bry.* chews.)
Dilated pupils: squinting and rolling eyes.
Fidgety feet.

MUMPS

PILOCARPUS MYCROPHYLLUS
(Jaborandi)

Dr. Burnett's homœopathic remedy for mumps seems to surpass all the rest, i.e. PILOCARPUS. It acts very quickly, and also relieves the pain.

Moreover, *Pilocarpus* has a reputation for the metastases in which mumps excels, whether to testes or mammae; when the swelling suddenly subsides, as the result of a chill, and worse troubles supervene. *Pilocarpus* also acts as a prophylatic.

ACONITUM NAPELLUS

For the *Acon.* fever with restlessness and anxiety.

BARYTA IODATA or MURIATICA

In the *Baryta* child: backward—shy—"deficient".

BELLADONNA

Inflammation of *right* parotid with bright redness and violent shooting pains.
Glowing redness of face. Sensitive to cold.

BROMIUM

Parotids, especially *left* affected: especially after scarlet fever.
"Swelling and hardness of left parotid: warm to touch."
Swelling of all glands about throat.
Slow inflammation of glands, with hardness.
Brom. especially helps those who are upset by being overheated:
   but when attack comes on, sensitive to colds and draughts.
Worse damp, hot weather.

CARBO VEGETABILIS

Parotitis. Face pale, cold. Involvement of mammae or testes.

MUMPS

LACHESIS MUTA

Especially *left* side parotid, enormously swollen: sensitive to least touch; least possible pressure—severe pain; shrinks away when approached: can scarcely swallow.

Throat sore internally. Face red and swollen. Eyes glassy and wild.

There is not the offensive mouth and dirty tongue of the *Mercs.*, but more throbbing; with the usual *Lachesis* horrible tension.

LYCOPODIUM

Begins *right* side, and goes to left.

It has not the offensive mouth and salivation of *Merc.*

Desires warm drinks.

MERCURIUS

Mumps, especially *right* side. Offensive salivation.

Foul tongue, and offensive sweat. (*Merc. corr.*)

PHYTOLACCA

Inflammation of sub-maxillary and *parotid* glands with stony hardness.

Pain shoots into ear when swallowing.

Worse cold and wet.

PULSATILLA

Lingering fever, or metastases (*Carbo veg.; Abrot.*).

If in mumps the patient gets a cold, the breasts swell in girls, the testicles in boys.

RHUS TOXICODENDRON

Parotid and sub-maxillary glands highly inflamed and enlarged.

Mumps on *left* side.

Worse cold: cold winds: cold wet.

"Always with herpes on lips."

SCARLET FEVER

Belladonna for scarlet fever affords an excellent example of homœopathy in the common cases of epidemic scarlet fever, and shows startling results, not only for the disease (when properly prescribed, i.e. when the symptoms agree), but also as a prophylactic.

Chief Remedy
BELLADONNA

Bright red, hot face. Glossy, scarlet skin: intense heat: "burns the hand."

"In the true Sydenham scarlet fever, where the eruption is perfectly smooth and truly scarlet."

Eyes red; injected: pupils later very dilated.

Lips—mouth—throat, red, dry, burning.

Strawberry tongue.

For eruptions like roseola and scarlet fever, with fever, sore throat, cough and headache.

Twitching, jerking; possibly wild delirium.

(*Apis* wants to be cool, uncovered: *Bell.* wants to be warm. *Bell.* also has more thirst.)

Cases where it has been used as a prophylatic, or used suitably on its indications, abort, or run a very mild course, leaving no sequelae, and are practically (as so many report), not even infectious.

Sequelæ

Hahnmeann wrote:

"*Belladonna* displays a valuable and specific power in removing the after-sufferings remaining from scarlet fever. . . . *Most medical men have hitherto regarded the consequences of scarlet fever as at least as dangerous as the fever itself and there have been many epidemics where more died of the after-effects than of the fever.*"

And he gives one interesting hint, "where ulceration has followed scarlet fever and where *Belladonna* is no longer of service," *Chamomilla* "will remove in a few days all tendency to ulceration: and the suffocating cough that sometimes follows the disease is also removed by *Chamomilla*, especially if accompanied by flushing of the face, and horripilation of limbs and back." (*Lesser Writings*.)

SCARLET FEVER

OTHER REMEDIES

AILANTHUS

Scarlet fever; plentiful eruption of bluish tint.
Eruption slow to appear, remains livid.
Irregular, patchy eruption of a very livid colour.
Throat livid, swollen, tonsils swollen with deep ulcers.
Pupils widely dilated (*Bell.*).
Semi-conscious, cannot comprehend.
Dizzy: can't sit up. Restless and anxious: later, insensible with muttering delirium.
Tongue dry, parched, cracked.
"Malignant scarlet fever."

AMMONIUM CARBONICUM

Malignant type (*Ail.*) with somnolence.
Body red, as if covered with rash.
Dark red and putrid throat. External throat swollen.
As if forehead would burst.
State like blood poisoning: great dyspnœa; face dusky and puffy.

APIS

Thick rose-coloured rash, feels rough. Or,
When rash does not come out, with great inflammation of throat, with scarlet fever in family.
Throat sore, swollen, œdematous: with stinging pain.
Convulsions when rash fails to come out (compare *Bry.*, *Cup.*, *Zinc.*, as given, under MEASLES).
Worse from heat: wants covers off: a cool room: (reverse of *Bell.*, wants warmth).

LACHESIS MUTA

Advanced stages: malignant scarlet fever.
Purple face.
Worse for heat (reverse of *Bell.*).
Bursting, hammering pains in head.
Throat worse left side: may extend to right.
Jealousy and suspicion suggests *Lach.*
Impelled to talk: loquacious delirium.
Lach. sleeps into an aggravation.

MERCURIUS

May follow *Bell.* for sore mouth, throat, tonsils, with ulceration and excessively foul breath.
Perspiration which aggravates the symptoms.

RHUS TOXICODENDRON

"Useful in scarlet fever with coarse rash. Or rash suppressed with inflammation of glands and sore throat" (KENT).

"You may rely on *Rhus* whenever acute diseases take on a typhoid form, as in scarlet fever, when no other remedy is positively indicated" (FARRINGTON).

"*Rhus* supplants *Bell*. when child grows drowsy and *restless*."

Fauces dark-red, with œdema (*Apis*).

Tongue red (? smooth) with triangular red tip.

TEREBINTHINA

Albuminuria and uræmia following scarlet fever.
Toxic: confused: better profuse urination.
Often indicated in dropsy after scarlet fever.
Hæmaturia: urine cloudy and smoky.
"Hæmaturia: dyspnœa: drowsiness."
Tongue dry and glossy.

N.B.—*Acidum nitricum*, *Phosphorus*, or one of many other drugs might be needed in difficult cases, or in cases first seen later on in the disease and with complications; according to the symptoms and make-up of the patient.

For SUPPRESSED or RECEDING eruption, see under MEASLES.

SMALL-POX

ACONITUM NAPELLUS
To modify first stage and early second stage.
High fever: great restlessness. Fear of death.

ANTHRACINUM
Gangrenous cases, with severe burning.

ANTIMONIUM TARTARICUM
Long held by homœopaths to be specific for small-pox.
Pustules with red areola, like small-pox, which leave a crust and form a scar.
Pains in back and loins.
Violent pain in sacro-lumbar region: slightest movement causes retching and cold sweat.
Violent headache: < evening; < lying; > sitting up; > cold.
Variola; backache, headache; cough with crushing weight on chest; before or at beginning of eruptive stage; diarrhœa, etc. Also when eruption fails.
LILIENTHAL says: "Tardy eruption with nausea, vomiting, sleeplessness, or suppression of eruption. Putrid variola with typhoid symptoms (*Bapt.*).

APIS
Erysipelatous redness and swelling, with stinging-burning pains, throat and skin.
Absence of thirst.
Urine scanty—later suppressed.

ARSENICUM ALBUM
Great sinking of strength.
Burning heat: frequent small pulse.
Great thirst. Great restlessness.
Rash irregularly developed with typhoid symptoms.
Hæmorrhagic cases, or when pustules sink in, and areolae grow livid.
Metastasis to mouth and throat.
Worse cold. (*Apis* worse heat.)

SMALL-POX

BAPTISIA

Typhoid symptoms: fœtid breath.
Pustules thick on arch of palate, tonsils, uvula, in nasal cavities; but scanty on skin.
Great prostration with pain in sacral region.
Drowsy; comatose; limbs feel "scattered".

BELLADONNA

First stage; high fever and cerebral congestion.
Intense swelling of skin and mucous membrane.
Dysuria and tenesmus of bladder.
Delirium and convulsions. Photophobia.

CROTALUS HORRIDUS

Pustular eruptions. After vaccination.
Eruptions, boils, pustules, gangrenous conditions, when fever is low and parts bluish.
Hæmorrhagic cases.

CUPRUM SULPHURICUM

Cerebral irritation, where eruption fails to appear. Convulsive phenomena.

HAMAMELIS VIRGINICUS

Hæmorrhagic cases oozing of dark blood from nose; bleeding gums; hæmatemesis, bloody stools.

HIPPOZÆNINUM
(Nosode of Glanders)

Low forms of malignant ulcerations, especially where nasal cartilages are affected.
Confluent small-pox.
Pustules and ulcers spread extensively over body till hardly a part remains free.

HYOSCYAMUS

Eruption fails to appear, causing great excitement, rage, anguish, delirium in paroxysms. Wants to get out of bed, and uncover.

LACHESIS MUTA

Hæmorrhagic cases.
Worse after sleep.
Dusky or purplish appearance, with excessive tenderness to touch.

MALANDRINUM

(The nosode of "grease"* in horses.)
CLARKE says: Homœopaths have found in *Maland.* a very effectual protection against infection with small-pox and vaccination.

MERCURIUS

Stage of maturation: ptyalism. Tendency of blood to head.
Moist swollen tongue with great thirst.
Diarrhœa or dysentery with tenesmus, especially during desiccation.

PHOSPHORICUM ACIDUM

Confluent, with typhoid conditions.
"Pustules fail to pustulate; degenerate into large blisters, which leave raw surface."
Stupid: wants nothing: not even a drink.
Answers questions but does not talk.
Subsultus tendinum: restlessness. Fear of death.
Watery diarrhœa.

PHOSPHORUS

Hæmorrhagic diathesis. Bloody pustules.
Hard dry cough: chest raw.
Hæmorrhage from lungs.
Back as if broken: faintings. Great thirst.

RHUS TOXICODENDRON

"Eruption turns livid and typhoid symptoms supervene."
Dry tongue. Sordes lips and teeth.
Wants to get out of bed. Great restlessness (*Ars.*).
Confluent: great swelling at first, afterwards eruption shrinks, and becomes livid.

---

* "*Grease*" *in horses was, or is believed to be identical with pustules occurring on the udders of cows, which affected the hands of milkmaids and rendered them immune from Small-pox: it was from this observation that inoculation and later vaccination (from* "*cow-pox*") *arose.*

SARRACENIA PURPUREA

(Drug of the North American Indians) seems to have done marvellous work in aborting and curing small-pox.

SULPHUR

Tendency to metastasis to brain during suppuration.

Stage of desiccation: or occasionally inter-current remedy where others fail.

THUJA

Which will cause the pustules of vaccination to wither and abort, should be one of the remedies of small-pox also.

LILIENTHAL says: "Pains in arms, fingers, hands, with fullness and soreness of throat.

"Areola round pustules marked and dark red.

"Pustules milky and flat, painful to touch. Give especially during stage of maturation, it may prevent pitting."

VARIOLINUM

Probably the most potent of all, having the complete picture of the disease from which it is prepared.

Dullness of head.

Severe pains in back and limbs, which became quite numb.

Chills, followed by high fever.

Violent headache.

White-coated tongue.

Great thirst.

Severe pains and distress in epigastric region with nausea and vomiting, mostly of greenish water.

In many cases profuse diarrhœa. In some, despondency.

Small-pox pustules on different parts of the body, mostly abdomen and back. Pustules perfectly formed, some umbilicated, some purulent.

"Given steadily the disease will run a milder course. It changes imperfect pustules into regular ones, which soon dry up. Promotes suppuration and desiccation. Prevents pitting" (LILIENTHAL).

TYPHOID AND TYPHOID CONDITIONS IN FEVERS

ARNICA

Says she is "So well!" when desperately ill.
Can be roused, answers correctly, then goes back into stupor (*Bapt., Phos. a.*).
"I am not sick: I did not send for you; go away!"
Foul breath—stool. Hæmorrhagic tendency.
"Bed feels so hard" (*Bapt., Pyrogen*).
"So sore", can only lie on one part a little time: restlessness *from this cause*.
Involuntary and unnoticed stools and urine.

ARSENICUM ALBUM

Rapid sinking of strength: great emaciation.
Least effort exhausts.
Great restlessness: constantly moves head and limbs: trunk still, because of extreme weakness. Tongue dry, brown, black.
Face distorted, hippocratic, sunken, anxious.
Rapid sinking of forces: extreme prostration.
ANXIETY: RESTLESSNESS: EXHAUSTION.
Thinks he must die. (*Arn.* says he is "not ill".)
Worse 1–2 a.m. and p.m.
Cadaveric aspect: cadaveric smelling stools.
Thirst for cold sips.

BAPTISIA

Typhoid fever. Typhoid conditions in fevers.
Rapid onset. Rapid course.
Abdomen distends early.
Odour horrible. Delirium.
Besotted condition: purple, bloated face.
Answers a word or two, and is back in stupor.
Feels there are two of him. Is scattered.
Tries to get the pieces together (*Pyrog.*).
In typhoid, "*Bapt.* vies with *Pyrog.* and *Arn.*"

BRYONIA ALBA

A most persistent remedy: develops slowly.
Lacerating, throbbing, jerking headache.
Nausea and disgust, whitish tongue.
Bitter taste. Thirst for large draughts of cold water (*Phos.*).
"Nervous, versatile or cerebral typhoid."
Sluggishness, then complete stupefaction.
When roused, is confused: sees images.
Thinks he is away from home and wants to be taken home.
Irrational talk: *prattles of his business:* worse after 3 p.m.
Delirium apt to start about 9 p.m.
Wants to be quiet. Pain, limbs, when moving.
Tongue dry.
Easily angered.
Faint if sits up.

CARBO VEGETABILIS

"A sheet-anchor in low states of typhoid, in the last stages of collapse; where there is coldness, cold sweat, great prostration; dyspnœa —wants to be fanned. Cold tongue."
"Desperate cases. Blood stagnates in the capillaries."
Blueness—coldness—ecchymoses.
Can hardly breathe, air-hunger. Says "Fan me! Fan me!"
Hæmorrhages, dark, decomposed, unclotted (*Crot. h.*).
Indescribable paleness face and body.

CROTALUS HORRIDUS

Typhoid with decomposition of blood and hæmorrhages—anywhere.
Intestinal hæmorrhage; blood dark, fluid, non-coagulable.
Tongue fiery-red, smooth, polished (*Pyrog.*), intensely swollen.
Yellowness of skin is an indication for *Crot. h.*
"*Lach.* cold and clammy: *Crot. h.* cold and dry."
Attacks that come on with great rapidity (*Bapt., Hyos.*).
Rapidly increasing unconsciousness. Besotted appearance (*Bapt.*).
Typhoid when it becomes putrid.
"Diseases of the very lowest, the most putrid type, coming on with unusual rapidity."

TYPHOID

HYOSCYAMUS

Fevers rapidly develop the typhoid state (*Bapt.*, *Crot. h.*).
Sensorium clouded.
Staring eyes: Carphology. Picks bedclothes.
Teeth covered with sordes.
Tongue dry, unwieldy, rattles in mouth, so dry.
Involuntary stool and urine (*Phos.*, *Arn.*).
Subsultus tendinum.
Mutters, or says no word for hours.
Mentally very suspicious: refuses medicine, thinks you will poison him (*Rhus.*, *Lach.*).
Jealous (*Lach.*). Alternately mild and timid, then violent. Will scratch, and try to injure.
Exposes person (*Phos.*). Wants to be naked.
Talks to imaginary people: to dead people.
Illusions: hallucinations; talking, with delirium, then stupor.
Early can be roused: later complete unconsciousness.

LACHESIS MUTA

Loquacity: delirium with great loquacity.
Face puffy, purple, mottled.
Much rumbling in distended abdomen.
Clothing cannot be tolerated: must not touch abdomen or throat.
Tongue swells (*Crot. h.*): difficult to protrude.
Suspicious. "Trying to poison her!" (*Rhus.*).
Worse after sleep: sleeps into aggravation.
Cold, clammy (*Crot. h.* cold, dry).
Stool with dark blood.

MURIATICUM ACIDUM

"Also one of our best remedies in typhoid."
Tongue dry, leathery, shrunken (*Hyos.*, *Ars.*).
Muscular prostration comes first, mind remains long clear (reverse of *Phos. acid*).
Lower jaw drops. Slides down in bed from excessive weakness (*Phos. acid*).
Cannot urinate without the bowels also moving.
"Nearer to *Carbo veg.* than any other remedy."

PHOSPHORICUM ACIDUM

"One of our best remedies in typhoid."
Simultaneous depression of animal, sensorial and mental life from the start.
Slowly increasing prostration.
Advanced typhoid.
Lies in stupor, unconscious of all that goes on: but if roused is fully conscious.
Glassy stare, as if slowly comprehending.
Prostration. Tympanitic abdomen.
Dry brown tongue. Dark lips. Sordes.
Bleeding; nose, lungs, bowels (*Crot. h.*).
Jaw drops: "as if must die of exhaustion."

PHOSPHORUS

Abdomen distended, sore, very sensitive to touch (*Lach.*).
Worse lying left side: better, right.
Stools offensive, bloody, involuntary. *The Anus appearing to remain open* (*Apis.*).
Burning in stomach: burning thirst for cold water. Desire for ice cream.
Fear alone: in the dark: of thunder.
Especially useful in typhoid pneumonias.
Suspicious (*Lach.*).

PYROGENIUM

(BURNETT's great remedy for typhoid.)
Bed feels hard (*Bapt.*).
Great restlessness: must constantly move (*Rhus*), to relieve soreness of parts (*Arn.*).
Tongue clean, smooth, fiery-red; or dry and cracked.
Horribly offensive diarrhœa (*Bapt.*).
Sense of duality (*Bapt.*).
Pulse quick: or out of proportion to temperature.

RHUS TOXICODENDRON

"Fevers take on the typhoid type: triangular red-tipped tongue and restlessness."
Cannot rest in any position (*Pyrog.*).
Slow and difficult mentation. May answer correctly. Talks to himself.
Refuses food and medicine. Fears poison (*Hyos.*, *Lach.*).
Dreams of strenuous exertion.

TARAXACUM

Restlessness of limbs wth tearing pain. "Like *Rhus* only *mapped tongue.*"

TEREBINTHINA

Tongue bright-red, smooth, glazed (*Pyrog.*).
Extreme tympanites (*Phos. acid.*, *Phos.*).
Thick scanty urine: mixed with blood, or cloudy, smoky, albuminous.
Diarrhœa with blood intermixed.
Fresh ecchymoses in great numbers (*Arn.*).

ILL-EFFECTS OF VACCINATION

Homœopathy has a very great *antidote to vaccination, and remedy for the after-effects of vaccination*, in THUJA.

Numbers of persons date their ill-health, their years of headache, asthma, epilepsy, etc., from vaccination. It is just the cases that do not "take" that seem more particularly liable to chronic ill-health.

THUJA

A direct antidote to the vaccinial poison.

In acute cases, wipes out the fever and eruption, and causes the pustules to disappear.

In chronic diseases, it may be impossible to cure many conditions without *Thuja*. Where symptoms improve to a point, and then always recur, while the disease can be traced back to a vaccination, or vaccinations, *Thuja* will generally supply the deep stimulus that leads to cure.

OTHER REMEDIES

ARNICA

Must not be forgotten. It does not destroy the vaccination like *Thuja* and *Maland.*, but it has amazing power of taking away pain, swelling, and general malaise, while the process goes on to completion.

MALANDRINUM

Nosode, prepared from "grease" in horses. Very like *Thuja* in symptoms and effects.

CLARKE says: "Burnett's indications are—Lower half of body: greasy skin and eruptions. Slow pustulation, never ending."

SILICA

The *Sil.* patient is feeble, lacks "grit", shrinks from responsibility. Is chilly: sensitive to draughts, but enervated with very hot weather. Head sweats at night. (*Calc.*) Sweaty, offensive feet.

SULPHUR

Warm patient. Hungry for everything: for fats.
Intolerant of clothing and weight of clothes.
Kicks off bedclothes: puts feet out. Eruptions of every kind.

WHOOPING-COUGH

ANTIMONIUM TARTARICUM
Cough when child gets angry, and after eating. Ends in vomiting. "Chest full of rattles." Thirstless: coated tongue.

ARNICA
"A wonderful whooping-cough remedy."
Violent tickling cough if child gets angry: *Begins to cry before cough* (*Bell.*): knows it is coming and dreads it.

BELLADONNA
Weeping and pains in stomach before coughing. Feels head will burst.
Dry spasmodic cough, worse at night; lying.
"Spasms of larynx which cause cough and difficulty of breathing" (KENT).
Kent says, "The *Bell.* cough is peculiar. As soon as great violence and great effort have raised a little mucus there is peace, during which larynx and trachea get dryer and dryer and begin to tickle, then comes the spasm and the whoop, and the gagging." Especially after exposure to cold.

BROMIUM
With sensation of coldness in throat.
Larynx as if covered with velvet, but feels cold.
"Whooping cough in spring, towards hot weather." Worse hot weather.

BRYONIA ALBA
"Child coughs immediately after eating and drinking and vomits, then returns to the table, finishes his meal, but coughs and vomits again" (LILIENTHAL).
"Dry spasmodic cough; whooping cough, shaking the whole body." Cough makes him spring up in bed—even *Bry.*

CARBO ANIMALIS
With feeling of coldness in chest.
Severe dry cough, shakes abdomen as if all would fall out; must support belly (*Dros.*).

CARBO VEGETABILIS

Cough, mostly hard and dry: or sounds rough: apt to occur after a full meal.

Every violent spell brings up a lump of phlegm, or is followed by retching, gagging and waterbrash.

Pain in chest after cough: burning as from a coal of fire.

Craving for salt. (This determined the remedy in a case that promptly recovered.)

"One of the greatest medicines we have in the beginning of whooping-cough. Gagging, vomiting and redness of face" (KENT).

Paroxysms of violent spasmodic coughing: with cold sweat and cold pinched face after attack.

CINA

Becomes rigid, with clucking sound down in oesophagus as paroxysm ends.

Not relieved by eating: stomach bloated, yet hungry. Grits teeth.

COCCUS CACTI

Worse at night, when hot in bed.

Better lying in cool room without much covering: wants room cold.

If mother can get to it quickly enough with a drink of cold water she can ward off the paroxysm.

Child holds its breath to prevent coughing.

"Wakes in morning with paroxysm of whooping-cough, which ends in vomiting ropy mucus, which hangs in long strings from mouth—great ropes. Here *Coccus c.* will cut short the disease." ("*Kali bi.* stringy but yellow: *Coccus c.* clear" or white.)

CORALLIUM RUBRUM

Smothered sensation before cough. Exhaustion after.

CUPRUM METALLICUM

Better by swallowing cold water.

Uninterrupted paroxysms till breath completely exhausted. Gasps with repeated crowing inspirations till black in the face. Mucus in trachea and spasms in larynx.

Cramps beginning in fingers and toes.

Thumbs tucked in during cough.

WHOOPING-COUGH

DROSERA

Impulses to cough follow one another so violently, that he can hardly get his breath.
Oppression of the chest, as if something kept back the air when he coughed and spoke, so that the breath could not be expelled.
When he breathes out a sudden contraction in hypogastrium makes him heave and excites coughing.
Crawling in larynx which provokes coughing.
On coughing he vomits water, mucus and food.
When coughing, contractive pain in the hypochondria. Cannot cough on account of the pain, unless he presses his hand on the pit of the stomach.
The region below the ribs is painful when touched and, when coughing, must press his hand on the spot to mitigate the pain.
Spasmodic cough, with retching and vomiting, caused by tickling or dryness in throat.

IPECACUANHA

Stiffens: goes rigid, loses breath: grows pale: then relaxes and vomits phlegm with relief.
Convulsions in whooping-cough, frightful spasms especially of left side.

KALI CARBONICUM

Convulsive and tickling cough at night.
Cough so violent as to cause vomiting.
Cough at 3 a.m., repeated every half-hour.
Bag-like swellings between the upper lids and the eyebrows; often puffy face also.
"Dry, hard, racking, hacking cough."

KALI SULPHURICUM

Whooping-cough, with retching, without vomiting. Yellow, slimy expectoration.
Tongue coated with yellow mucus.
Hot and sweating. *Hates* cough and weeps. (*Bell.*)
Looks "fair, fat and forty" even a child.

LOBELIA

Cough ends with violent sneezing.

WHOOPING-COUGH

MAGNESIA PHOSPHORICA

Violent spasmodic attacks of cough, with face blue and turgid. Ends in a whoop.

MEPHITIS

Whooping or any violent cough: very violent, spasmodic, as if each spell would terminate life.
Frequent paroxysms especially at night.
Desire for salt (*Carbo veg.*).
Worse lying down. Child must be raised.